Body Lotions For Beginners

BY LINDSEY PYLARINOS

The Ultimate Guide to Making All Natural Body Lotions for Glowing, Youthful, Vibrant Skin

2nd Edition

Table Of Contents

Introduction

I want to thank you and congratulate you for purchasing the book, "Body Lotions for Beginners: The Ultimate Guide to Making All Natural Body Lotions for Glowing, Youthful, Vibrant Skin."

This book contains proven steps and strategies on how to make all natural body lotions.

Making lotion is not as simple as you may have thought it is. You need to know the properties and purpose of each ingredient in making lotion. The first part of the book discusses the ingredients and equipment needed in making lotion while the later part of the book provides the step by step method in making lotion.

Thanks again for purchasing this book, I hope you enjoy it!

Chapter 1 – Body Lotions

The skin is more than just the covering of our body. It is the body's largest organ, and it has important roles in ensuring the healthy functioning of the entire body. One of the skin's major attributes is that it is semi-permeable. Because of this feature, certain substances can penetrate the skin while other substances are blocked. Therefore, the skin both protects and nourishes the body. To explain, several toxins are sweated out through the skin and there are lots of nutrients that are absorbed in the body through the skin. Bacteria are blocked from entry in the body, and essential body fluids are contained.

This fact indicates that what you apply to your face and skin is as essential as what you eat. In other words, natural cosmetics are as good as the natural food you eat. Most of the ingredients used in making natural products for your skin are usually found in your kitchen while other ingredients can be purchased from specialty shops selling natural, organic products. The recipes in this book use only organic plant based ingredients.

In order to keep the skin supple and in good condition, effective skin care is needed so it will look beautiful and carry out its function perfectly. Using natural substances like essential oils, fruits, flower waters, honey and others in homemade lotions can provide different skin treatments for all types of skin. The body lotion recipes in this ebook are easy to make and are all natural and healthy. They are also cheaper than the commercially available lotion that you would normally buy. Furthermore, you can experiment with and test other skin care ideas.

The ingredients used for making your own body lotions are known to be safe, effective and beneficial to your skin. A body lotion is a topical preparation used as a moisturizer to prevent or treat rough, dry, itchy, scaly skin and some minor skin irritations. Lotions are types of emollients that soften and moisturize the skin as well as reduce the flaking and itching. Lotions may be applied to the skin using a clean cloth, a brush, cotton wool, gauze or even just your bare hands. There are lots of lotions, particularly hand and body lotions, that are formulated not as a medicine, but as means to re-hydrate, soften and smoothen the skin.

Chapter 2 – Basic Ingredients and Equipment Used in Making Natural Body Lotions

There are lots of commercial lotions that claim to soften and enhance the skin, but they actually contain harmful chemicals and synthetic fragrances that may irritate the body. Finding a body lotion that you like that does not contain any harmful ingredients can be difficult as these are often expensive. Body lotions are supposed to help the skin and not damage it. Save your skin and money by creating your own natural body lotion that is effective not only for your body but for your face as well. What you apply on your body has a great effect on your health just as what you eat may affect your body too.

A good lotion can likewise boost your spirits with the help of aromatherapy. You can customize your recipe using the essential oils that you like. There are some ingredients for natural body lotions that you might not be familiar with, though you can find a number of them in your local health store. Natural body lotions contain natural ingredients. Each ingredient has its own function and purpose.

Ingredients

Preservatives

Preservatives are vital if you intend to give your lotion to someone as a gift or to sell it. German Plus is the most popular type of preservative that is easy to use because it is a paraben-free preservative, but there are lots of them available in the market.

Honey

Honey is very effective for softening and healing skin, and it has been utilized successfully to treat minor burns. It is a natural humectant, which means it attracts and retains moisture. The antioxidant and natural hydrating properties of honey trap and keep moisture, cleanse complexion and rejuvenate the skin, leaving the skin soft. Honey in its purest form is perfect for all types of skin, and has great holistic healing properties.

Honey is considered as one of the greatest gifts of nature. It is not only healthy when consumed, but is very helpful in keeping the skin healthy. Its medicinal and beauty benefits have been popular to humankind for centuries. There are some stories that the Ancient Egyptian queen Cleopatra used honey and milk whenever she bathed. She also used milk and honey as facial lotion. At present, honey is used as a vital skin care ingredient by cosmetic companies to help with different skin conditions.

Honey is an effective moisturizer. It has humectant properties so it is used as a moisturizer in many cosmetic preparations including lotions. It does not only attract water, but also retains it in the skin, thus keeping the skin elastic and supple. It likewise protects against dryness and wrinkles.

Lemon

Lemon is a gentle skin bleach, which helps remove age spots and freckles. This fruit has a wonderful fragrance, and is added to beverages and beauty products. The fruit is high in vitamin C, with anti-bacterial effects and anti-carcinogenic and antioxidant properties. The juice consists of around 5% acid, making it very useful for different household purposes.

Cetyl Alcohol

Thickens and stabilizes your lotion and makes your lotion glidy. The higher the amount of thicker, the more moisturizing your lotion will be.

Distilled or Deionzed Water

Your lotion usually contains 55%-80% water. The more water, the thinner your lotion will be. Add an extra 10% because you will lose some water through evaporation.

Essential Oils

Essential oils have been used consistently in beauty and skin care treatments from the time of their discovery. There are lots of benefits in using organic and natural essential oils in your home made lotions. Essential oils speed up the removal of old skin cells and stimulate the growth of new skin cells. These oils reduce inflammation and control the production of sebum, and most of all their wonderful smell is soothing and calming, reducing stress and aiding in relaxation. Some essential oils have a rejuvenating effect on the skin and they help to keep you looking and feeling beautiful and young.

Beeswax

Beeswax acts as a surfactant when combined with cold creams and other skin lotion, forming a protective barrier on the skin. It adds body to skin care products, which makes creams thicker. Unlike royal jelly and honey, beeswax has anti-inflammatory, antiviral and antibacterial benefits which make it ideal in healing minor skin irritations. The substance acts as a humectant and an emollient that attracts moisture to the skin and seals it in. The substance has vitamin A, which is effective in softening and rehydrating dry skin. Beeswax improves the consistency of lotions.

Equipment

Some of the equipment used in making soap is also used in making lotion. The process in making natural homemade body lotions is easy and fast. Just make sure that you have all the ingredients and the needed equipment ready.

1. Saucepan – it is used in melting the solid ingredients. Others suggest using a double broiler for a safer method of melting.

2. Measuring tools – used in measuring the ingredients accurately. This may include measuring cups and measuring spoons.

3. Large glass bowl – used in mixing the ingredients

4. Mixer - it is best to use a wood hand mixer so the mixture will not stick on the mixer.

5. Spatula

6. Container – it should be a 16 oz wide mouth glass jar, a recycled honey bottle or other container similar to this.

7. Stick Blender – preferably stainless steel. You will use this in whisking. If you are making a small amount of lotion, a strong arm is enough to whisk the mixture.

8. Digital thermometer – if you don't have one, you can use a glass candy thermometer

9. Digital scale – for weighing your lotion

Don't forget to sterilize these tools and equipment before making the lotion. Bacteria might be present and may cause deterioration of your mixture.

Chapter 3 – Basic Instructions in Making Lotion

As defined in Chapter 1, lotion is the emulsification of water and oil by means of some kind of waxy agent. These days, there are lots of people who prefer to create their own lotion instead of buying one. One of the primary benefits of making your own natural lotion is that you are sure that the ingredients in making it are all natural and do not contain any harmful chemicals. Next, is that you can customize your lotion. For example, if you want an all natural honey lotion with some essential oils, you can have it instantly.

Here are the basic instructions in making a lotion. Keep in mind that there are lots of instructions given online, but most of them do not provide the right consistency and pH of your lotion. The instruction involves two methods – Method 1 which is the Quick and Easy method and Method 2 the Mixing of all the Ingredients.

Method 1 – The Quick and Easy Method

Every lotion is somewhat different and you will never go wrong when making it. The purpose of each ingredient in making the lotion was mentioned in the previous chapter.

2-3 tbsp (30-45 g) distilled water or aloe vera gel
2 tbsp (30 g) beeswax
Essential oil(s) (a few drops)
1/2 cup (4 oz) grapeseed oil or jojoba, or coconut
Vitamin E oil or capsule

In a saucepan under low heat, melt the beeswax, vitamin E oil and the grapeseed oil. You should mix it slowly – you don't want to burn your materials. The secret for a better product is to be patient. Using a double boiler is a good idea. If you can afford to buy one, then do so as using this is the safest way of melting your ingredients.

When the ingredients are melted entirely, remove them from the heat. Transfer the mixture into a big glass bowl right away. Otherwise, if the mixture overcooks, it will not form. After transferring the solution, clean the pan with soap and water. Soak it right away.

Add the aloe vera gel or water. If you want a thicker, butter-like consistency, reduce the amount of water. Use a hand mixer in mixing. Mix until your scented mixture becomes thick. You can replace distilled water with rose water if that is the scent that you want to achieve. You can purchase rose water from your local grocery store.

Let it sit for 15 to 20 minutes. It requires time to thicken up and gel. There is no need for you to transfer it in a cold area – just leave it on the counter and wait for several minutes.

As the time passes and your lotion has formed, scoop it out into a glass jar or any other container ideal for lotion. Label it and wrap it up to customize it.

Method 2 – Mixing all the Ingredients

Prepare the ingredients and equipment as needed. With this method you can add/remove/substitute ingredients. This method will make use of the following ingredients:

1/8 teaspoon (dash) rosemary extract or vitamin E oil

22 oz aloe vera gel or distilled water
1 tea bag of your choice
5 oz scented oil
1/2 tsp cinnamon
1 tsp (5 g) each of selected herbs
1 tbsp (15 g) stearic acid
5 tbsps (75 g) emulsifying wax or shredded beeswax
1/2 tsp (pinch) citric acid
1 tsp honey
1/2 tsp potassium sorbate

Boil the distilled water or aloe vera gel/juice. Once there is enough bubbling, lower the heat to medium. Add the citric acid, potassium sorbate and cinnamon. Once dissolved, add 1 tbsp each of the herbs you choose and one tea bag of your choice. After everything has been simmered for 10 minutes on medium to low heat, continue simmering for another 30 minutes.

The next step is to work on your oil mixture. Using a small pan or pot, add 5 oz of your preferred essential oil mixed with 5 tbsps emulsifying wax or beeswax, 1 tbsp stearic acid, 1 tsp of honey and approximately 1/8 tsp vitamin E oil or rosemary extract.

Once the herb mixture has finished, boil water in a medium pot. You can use the bottom of your double boiler alternately. In a large mixing bowl, strain the herb mixture, squeeze all the good juice out of the tea bag and herbs.

Add all the ingredients in the bowl. Once the water is boiling, set the small pot of oils on top until the wax is dissolved. Make sure that you will not overcook it. Stir it and don't allow the oil to get too hot – that is the purpose of the double boiler. When it reaches this point, remove it from heat immediately.

This step normally takes time, but you need to keep an eye on the bowl. It is best if you remain there to stir and make sure that nothing will go wrong.

Beat the herb mixture as you add the oil mixture. Be very careful as this stuff may burn. It's ok to let the mixture cool down a little, but there is no need for the mixture to be hot to be able to mix it. Blend on medium heat for two minutes.

You can use the blender in mixing it, but it is not recommended since the blender will not function the same afterwards.

Continue mixing and stirring using a rubber spatula to get all the air bubbles out. Add one drop of fragrance or essential oil for two ounces of total mixture. The mixture will be watery until it cools and sets, so don't panic if it looks runny.

Let it stand for two hours before transferring the mixture in the bottles. If you will be using a plastic container, make sure that it is not too hot and it will still have lots of air bubbles. Make use of a turkey baster or funnel baster for easy pouring.

Refrigerate your homemade natural lotion until it is time to use it. Your lotion will last up to three months under room temperature. Don't leave it in direct sunlight.

Lotion recipes are made to be perfect. If you are not 100% happy with this recipe, continue tweaking until you have a recipe this unique to you.

What You Need to Keep in Mind When Making Lotion

> Make sure the water and oil are hot, but not too hot. They should be at the same temperature when mixing.

> The less water, the longer your mixture will last. You can use a strong antioxidant aloe vera or tea as your water. You can also use distilled water and let it boil before adding to it.

> Citric acid and potassium sorbate work well at 0.3% and together with a pinch of cinnamon. Dissolve both ingredients at the beginning.

> Always add either Rosemary extract at 0.3% or Vitamin E at 0.5%, but not both, to the oil mixture to prevent the oil from being rancid and changing your lotion into yellow.

> Never use more than 30% oil unless you prefer the greasy or shiny after look.

> Xanthan gum, lecithin powder or stearic acid can be used at one to two percent to thicken. These ingredients are added to the oil mixture until dissolved.

> Use 1 tbsp wax or emulsifier per oz of oil. Melt into the oil mixture.

> When adding herbs into the oil, allow them to simmer for at least three hours.

> If you will add herbs in water, allow them to simmer for at least thirty to forty five minutes.

➢ Keep everything as sterile as possible.

➢ Honey is added to oil at one percent if desired. It is good for the skin and it will help in preserving the lotion.

➢ In using fragrance and essential oils, you usually don't need more than one drop per 2 oz.

➢ Use blueberry, citrus teas, rose petals, or raspberry for fragrance or color if you need your lotion to last long. Berries, other teas and other flower petals work well in quick blends that may only last for a week or so.

➢ Your blend should be at room temperature before transferring it to its containers.

The Do's and Don't's in Making Lotion

➢ Don't use food coloring or crayons. They are toxic. Flowers, tea, herbs and berries are excellent, natural colorants.

➢ Don't use toxic ingredients in making your homemade lotion. People have sensitive skin and products such as lotion usually stay on the skin without being washed off. Toxins go directly into the body, cells and bloodstream.

➢ Do not use a microwave in making your lotion. This appliance changes the molecular structure of your ingredients, thus rendering your lotion not as beneficial to your skin as it should be.

➢ Always test the product on a small area of your skin before using it on your entire body. It is best to check first whether or not you are allergic to some ingredients.

➢ Do not use cinnamon oil as it can irritate the skin. Used powdered cinnamon instead.

➢ Do not use lotion while it is still hot as it might burn your skin.

Chapter 4 – Homemade Body Lotion Recipes

Making your own homemade body lotion is a great way to take care of yourself. You will be able to save money and you are sure that you will be using natural and healthy products for your skin. The following recipes use natural skin moisturizers to heal, nourish and support your skin. As mentioned in Chapter 2 around 60% of what you apply to your skin is absorbed in your body, so using only natural ingredients in your homemade body lotion really helps a lot in improving your health.

Essential oils in lotion can do more than just protect and keep your skin healthy. It also makes your skin smoother and glowing when you use homemade lotion recipes. These oils also lift your mood, and calm your nerves and strengthen your immune system and also you will smell great.

Recipe in Making Unscented Homemade Lotion

Ingredients
1 tsp (5ml) Vitamin E
10 drops Grapefruit Seed extract (natural preservative)
1 to 2 tbsp (25ml) Vegetable Glycerin (optional)
10 to 20 drops Essential Oil (optional)
2 to 2 1/2 tbsp (3 to 8g) Emulsifying wax (depending on how thick you want it)
1/2 cup (125ml) distilled Water
1/2 tsp (2g) Stearic Acid (stabilizer derived from plant oils)
1/3 cup (75ml) Carrier Oil

Directions

1. Stir together the stearic acid, glycerin, oil, and emulsifying wax in the upper part of a double boiler,

heating slowly over a low heat until the wax is melted. Remove from heat and add the vitamin E.

2. Put another pot in the microwave or on the stove, gently warm the water until lukewarm.

3. Pour the water into the oil slowly, stir briskly with a whisk until you have a uniform color mixture.

4. Add in the essential oils as well as the grapefruit seed extract. Add the homemade body lotion in a clean, sterilized 8 oz PET plastic or dark glass bottle and let it cool before covering it.

5. The water and oil components of the lotion will separate as it cools down. To re-mix the lotion, shake it every ten to twenty minutes. As soon as the lotion cooled down completely, they will stay mixed.

6. Keep it in a cool, dark place.

Using Carrier Oils for Your Natural Homemade Lotion Recipes

You can add these aromatherapy carrier oils specific for each skin type. You can use one or you can combine oils to create the best mixture for your skin. Here is a sample guide to help you out when adding carrier oils in your homemade lotion. There are some carrier oils that you should only up to 10% of a recipe.

List of Carrier oils and its specific purpose:

Type of skin :Carrier Oils

Acne- prone, oily skin: Jojoba, grapeseed, neem

Aging, dry, damaged ski Avocado, calendula, olive, rosehip,sweet almond, sea buckthorn, borage, St. John's wort

Normal, combination :apricot kernel, sunflower, sweet almond, jojoba

Sensitive:calendula, rice bran, avocado, grapeseed, apricot kernel, kukui nut

Psoriasis, Eczema:sweet almond, jojoba, olive, Calendula, sea buckthorn, avocado, evening primrose, kukui nut,castor, rosehip, neem

Stretch Marks, Scars:Jojoba, rosehip, castor, sea buckthorm, Calendula, kukui nut

Using Essential Oils for your Natural Homemade Lotion Recipes

Below is a list of essential oils for each skin type. Select a few essential oils and add up to 20 drops per recipe. If you will be going out in the sunshine, do not use citrus essential oils like lemon, grapefruit, orange and bergamot. Citrus oils can increase your risk of sunburn.

Type of Skin: Essential Oils

Acne-prone, oily skin :Grapefruit, lemongrass, Bergamot, jasmine, geranium, juniper, lemon, patchouli, tea tree, cedarwood, ylang ylang, petitgrain

Aging,   Dry,   damaged:frankincense, peppermint,helichrysum,chamomile, patchouli, palmarosa, sandalwood, rose, ylang ylang

Normal, combination:Lavender, ylang ylang, geranium, palmarosa, jasmine, neroli

Sensitive:Lavender, rose, chamomile, jasmine, helichrysum, neroli, palmarosa

Psoriasis, eczema:Frankincense, patchouli, lavender, chamomile, helichrysum, sandalwood, palmarosa, rose

Stretch marks, scars:neroli, rosemary, helichrysum, rose, lavender, geranium, patchouli

Chapter 5 – Benefits of Adding Essential Oils in your Homemade Lotion

Essential oils can benefit different skin types and can penetrate into the deeper levels of your skin to develop new skin cells. Here are eight popular essential oils that you can add in your lotion as well as their benefits.

Bergamot

One of the top essential oils for skin is bergamot. This essential oil is also used in some of your favorite perfumes. It is not only a fragrant oil; it has many benefits for your skin. It has an antiviral properties that can help fight cold sores and reduce acne, bacteria and oil on your skin.

Rose

Rose oil is perfect for aging or sensitive skin. This type of oil is expensive and is hard to find. It has astringent properties that help in repairing broken capillaries and enhance the overall condition of the skin. It also helps in lightening the scars, stretch marks and acne marks and ease common symptoms of PMS.

Clary Sage

Clargy sage decreases inflammation, balances the skin's oil production and revitalizes the skin. It likewise helps ease pain from your monthly menstrual period and childbirth and helps you relax, so it is best to keep it around during that time of the month.

Geranium

To reap the benefits of geranium, you don't need a green thumb. This multi-purpose essential oil can do a multitude of wonders, such as eliminating body odor, promoting cell growth, causing ugly scars and spots to fade, and healing wounds on your skin. It has a flowery and calming scent that is perfect for helping you unwind.

Jasmine

This essential oil can soften and smoothen the skin. It helps you get in the mood for romance. You can use this oil in the bedroom and for getting rid of the scars and marks on your skin. The scent of the oil can make your skin clear from any blemishes and smell fresh as a flower.

Rosehip

If you are looking for a unique skin care oil, rosehip oil is what you need. This essential oil has Omega 3, 6, and 9, linoleic acids, lycopene and vitamin C. All of these elements help minimize the signs of aging, help regenerate skin cells, reduce fine lines, and moisturize and boost collagen that leaves the skin feeling soft and pampered.

Sandalwood

This essential oil has been used since Biblical times because of its healing properties. It is now being used as a calmative agent, reducing scars, reducing lines, and reviving tired, dull skin. You can likewise use this oil on your skin to restore moisture and shine.

Eucalyptus

You might not believe it, but eucalyptus has lots of benefits for your skin. It works the same way like tea tree oil, where it can help in getting rid of your acne, but it is likewise very effective in relieving headache. The anti-bacterial and anti-microbial effect of this oil can help relieve irritation, swelling, and redness of the acne.

The good thing about these essential oils is that you can use them on many other things aside from being a skin care oil. Don't forget to test oils before applying to your skin and in case you have sensitive skin, consult your dermatologist before trying them out.

Chapter 6 – Safety Colorants for Lotion

Colorants are ingredients that are used alone or in combination with other ingredients to alter the color of the lotion. These are used to make the product appealing and attractive, and for food to make it look appetizing. The colorants are also used to create a production image or specification, the product mood or other impression.

All the colorants used in cosmetics and other personal care products must be pre-approved by the Food and Drug Administration. The FDA performs safety reviews for colors used in cosmetics and the approval process may involve several studies to establish safety. The FDA lists the approved colors in the Code of Federal Regulations. The regulations describe the identity of the colors, the uses, restrictions, the allowed composition and any other requirement needed to make sure that they are using safe colorants.

The FDA has a regulatory body that checks on the color additives used in cosmetics, drugs, and food. The color additives used in cosmetics, particularly in lotion, should comply with the individual listing regulations issued by the FDA.

The use of an unlisted color additive or a color additive that does not conform to the identity and purity specifications of the listing regulations is not allowed. Most of the products contain a small amount of colorants.

Types of Colorants

Colorants are classified as either inorganic or organic depending on the chemistry. Originally, the organic colorants were called coal tar because the substances were derived from coal sources. However, these days all organic colorants are synthetic and are available as either oil soluble, insoluble or water soluble agents in all types of shades. Colorants are designated as FD&C, D&C or Ext. D&C. FD&C is certified for use in drugs, cosmetics and food.

Inorganic colorants include insoluble metallic compounds which are either derived from the natural resources or are synthesized. Compared to organic colorants, inorganic colorants do not have the same kinds of health risks and thus do not require certification.

Products that do not come into contact with the eyes or mucous membranes such as lotion, conditioner, shampoo, and hand cream use FD&C, Ext. D & C or D&C colors. Lotion uses a water soluble FD&C or D&C colors. Aside from the inorganic colors, there are other colorants which can be used in cosmetics. A small amount of colorant is enough to have the needed color for the lotion. Use only a small amount of colorant. Make sure that the color you use will complement the ingredients you used in your lotion. For instance, if you added rosehip essential oil, it would not be right to use green colorant as it will only cause confusion for the buyer/user.

Chapter 7: Adding Natural Preservatives to Increase Shelf Life

One way of keeping your skin vibrant and young looking is the daily application of natural homemade body lotion. Depending on the weather and your skin condition, application of body lotion can be done several times in a day. If you would religiously follow this routine, you could consume a regular sized bottle of lotion in a month's time. A shelf life of less than three months is therefore considered safe already. However, if you intend to give your homemade body lotions as gifts to friends or sell them for profit, then three to six months shelf life is ideal to ensure that the lotion is fresh and safe to use by the time they decide to use it (or at least, within a reasonable time frame).

You may wonder how come commercially prepared lotions could last for years. This is due to various chemicals and preservatives being added to the lotions. However, some of these ingredients are found to be harmful to the skin. That is why making your own lotion is safer and better for you. You know exactly what your lotion is made of.

How can you increase the shelf life of your homemade lotion?

Homemade lotions, devoid of toxic preservatives, are usually good for three months if placed in a dry, dim place with a cool temperature. If you live in a country with a warm climate, putting your lotion in the refrigerator would ensure prolonged shelf life, as bacteria tend to thrive and multiply in warm temperature. Sterile techniques of preparation should be strictly observed during the actual making of the lotion also so that contamination from bacteria could be prevented, thereby increasing its shelf life.

Another way of increasing the shelf life of your all-natural body lotion is to add natural preservatives to it. Unlike those preservatives in the commercially prepared skin products, these are safe and free from toxic and harsh properties. There are many available and proven natural preservatives that you can add to your lotion recipe. Before you decide which natural preservative to use, here are some tips.

➢ Although they are already considered as "natural", some preservatives can still trigger skin reactions or sensitivities to some people. This is not unusual as these preservatives contain antimicrobial, antifungal, or antibacterial properties that some people with sensitive skin cannot tolerate. One tip is not to put too much of these natural preservatives. Make sure also that you are not allergic or sensitive to these ingredients before you add them. Also, if you are planning to give your lotions as gifts to your friends or if you are planning to sell them, indicate all the added natural preservatives on the label.

➢ One problem usually encountered with adding preservatives is the difficulty in blending the odor. The undesirable odors of these natural preservatives can affect the overall smell of the finished product of the body lotions. It sometimes takes several tries or experiments before one can achieve the perfect amount to add in to the lotions while increasing their shelf life. The trick is to write down what you are doing while making the lotion. This way, when you achieve the goal of longer shelf life plus the right smell, consistency, color, and feel of the lotion, you have the exact formula that you can follow. You would be able to repeat it effortlessly.

➢ Avoid "doubling". This is when you put a preservative with a certain property, for instance, antibacterial property and then you add another preservative with the same property. This could only lead to a lotion that is too strong for the skin and might cause reactions or sensitivities.

➢ When preparing and handling the raw form of these preservatives, observe safety precautions as most of them can cause irritation to the eyes, skin, and respiratory system. You can provide protection by observing the following:

  o Make sure that little children and pets have no access to your working area. After making the lotion, secure the remaining preservatives by sealing the containers tightly and placing them in a cool, dry place, out of reach by children.
  o Wear protective apparel such as laboratory gown, disposable gloves, facemask, and eye goggles.
  o Avoid inhaling the ingredients as they can irritate the nasal lining and other parts of the respiratory system.
  o Ensure that no powder or droplets would get into your eyes. In the event that such happens, simply wash or flush your eyes with cool, clean, running water. Avoid scratching your eyes. If irritation persists, consult your doctor.
  o Do not let the ingredients have direct contact to your bare skin. Be extra careful when you have wounds or existing skin conditions. Again, simply flush with water if the ingredients accidentally come in contact with your skin or see your doctor if this does not work.

o Have paraphernalia or supplies exclusive for lotion making only. Do not use these utensils to other things, most especially when preparing your meals.

What are the best natural preservatives that you can use?

Here are some of the recommended natural preservatives that you can use to make your homemade lotion last longer, preferably till six months. These are usually available in your local stores or online suppliers.

1. Cinnamon. It is known to slow the growth of fungi, molds, yeast and some bacteria. According to some studies, combining cinnamon with potassium sorbate makes it a better preservative. Simply put a dash or up till ¼ teaspoon of this preservative to 16 ounces of the lotion. Take note however that cinnamon oil can be irritating to the skin, even if the dose is low. You might want to use the regular powder instead and just add water or oil mixture. Cinnamon is commonly found in the local grocery stores but if you prefer the top quality cinnamon products, you could acquire them from organic suppliers online.

2. Geranium Essential oil. This preservative can perform many tasks like fight off bacteria, inhibit growth of yeast, mold, fungi, and some bacteria plus it is also an antioxidant. Another strong point is that it has a great smell that could blend in wonderfully in your lotion, unlike most of the preservatives, which have undesirable smells. However, many describe the smell as feminine and this might not suit your male friends. It is also safe to use with other preservatives. You should add this last in your recipe. After the lotion is blended and when you are already in the final mixing, simply

add one drop of geranium essential oil to every 2 ounces of your homemade lotion. Again, you can purchase a quality product from your online organic supplier.

3. Citric Acid Powder. Aside from being an antioxidant and an effective preservative, citric acid powder is also used because of the following reasons:
    a. Prevention of rancidity and bacterial growth
    b. Adjustment of pH
    c. To stabilize color and ingredient of the lotion
To add the citric acid powder to your lotion, this is what you should do. First, boil the distilled water. Dissolve the citric acid powder, which is around .03% to .05% of the total amount of the distilled water. Set aside to cool. Add this to the homemade lotion. Take note, however, that if you plan to use your lotion as a sunscreen, do not add any citrus products.

4. Grapefruit Seed Extract (GSE) – Just like the first three preservatives, GSE helps control the growth of yeast, fungi, molds and some bacteria. It is soluble in water. The pH of GSE is at 2.5. In pure form, this preservative is very irritating to the skin. Wearing of gloves and extra caution is advised when handling this ingredient. Wearing of eye goggles is also advantageous for you. Make sure that it will not come in contact with broken skins. Even with this precaution, GSE has remained as one of the most popular preservatives among lotion makers. To the total lotion, just add 0.5% to 1% of GSE.

5. Potassium Sorbate. – it is known as the only preservative that is regarded as safe by the FDA. This is because for centuries of being used, there are very rare reports of any allergic reactions or toxic effects. It is non-irritating to the skin and works best when

combined with cinnamon. Still, when in its pure form, you should be very careful in handling this. Potassium sorbate is water soluble. Usage rate is at 0.1% to 0.5% only. Do not exceed this amount. The pH is preferably at 5-6. To keep the pH low, combine it with citric acid.

6. Green Tea Extract – This water-soluble preservative is known for being a strong antioxidant. It is known to be effective in fighting the occurrence of skin cancer and sun damage. In addition, skin regeneration is achieved because of this preservative. You can buy the gel caps and just break the cap to get the fluid inside. Add to your water mixture. Do not use more than 3%. A milder form of this is having green tea bags soak in the distilled water together with the citric acid. Let it cool. This technique has many benefits but the shelf life is lesser.

7. Benzoin Powder – aside from being an antioxidant, this preservative is also helpful in inhibiting the growth and proliferation of bacteria. It is not water-soluble. You need tinctures of alcohol to dissolve this product. Or you can add it to your oil raw when you are in the melting process. After that, strain the grits with a cheese cloth or a tight strainer. A lot of people use this. However, caution is also advised because it can be harmful to the skin. Do not add more than 0.25% of benzoin powder to your lotion. Also, be careful that you do not inhale, get it into your eyes, or come in contact with bare skin or wounds. It is known as a common skin irritant especially in its raw form.

8. Rosemary Oil Extract (ROE) – This preservative is also a natural antioxidant. It has a greenish tint that could

work well with your colorants to give your lotion that cool look. In your oil mixture, pour ROE at 0.1% to 0.5% only. Add this oil mixture to your lotion at one drop per ounce only. You can also opt for the Rosemary Extract powder. Use around 0.3% or about ¼ teaspoon for every 16 ounces of lotion.

9. Vitamin E T-50 or Vitamin E Mixed Tocopherol Oil – Although T-50 is not an organic product, it can be used with organic products. Vitamin E T-50 is usually used when Rosemary preservatives are not available. This preservative is used for the following reasons:
   a. Antioxidant.
   b. Protects oil from rancidity.
   c. Preserves the smell of the lotion.

Add 0.04 to 0.5% of this preservative to your lotion.

It may take several experiments before you finally discover which preservative works best for your homemade lotion. In the long run though, it would be advantageous to you as the shelf life of your lotion is increased in return.

Chapter 8: Turn Your Homemade Lotion Into A Sunscreen

Lotions have many purposes and one of them is your protection against skin damage from the sun, in the form of sunscreen. The sunlight, from 10 am to 3pm, has two types of rays that can cause harm to the skin. These are the UVA or the long wave ultraviolet A (which can cause aging of the skin) and the UVB or the short wave ultraviolet B (which can burn the skin).

You can maintain healthy, glowing, youthful, and vibrant skin when you use sunscreen every time you would be exposed to the sun for a long period of time. Commercially sunscreen products are not only expensive but they usually contain many ingredients that can be toxic to your skin too especially if you have sensitive skin. Hence, the ideal solution is turning your homemade lotion into sunscreen.

There are two types of sunscreens that you can add to your homemade lotion to convert them as sun block lotions. These are physical blocker sunscreen and chemical blocker sunscreen.

Physical blockers work by coating your skin with zinc oxide or titanium dioxide, blocking UVA and UVB radiation. On the other hand, chemical blockers, with the use of menthyl anthranilate, avobenzone, and benzophenones, would absorb UVA and UVB, thereby preventing sunburns. Unfortunately, it has been found out that chemical blockers can increase the risk of having skin cancer so the best option to use is the physical blockers.

Take note however, that some physical blockers can be carcinogenic (cancer-causing), too. For instance, titanium dioxide is said to be toxic and carcinogenic. The better choice is zinc oxide. However, not all zinc oxides are created equal. Nano-sized zinc oxide is made up of particles that are so tiny which means they can be absorbed by the skin, causing unintentional absorption of heavy metals into your body.

In choosing zinc oxide as a physical blocker to your lotion, make sure that you check the size. Non-nano sized zinc oxide is the best choice as it is too large and therefore cannot penetrate through your skin. You can get quality non-nano sized zinc oxide from suppliers online.

How to have economical, safe and effective sunscreen lotion

You can experiment and add the physical blockers to your homemade lotion recipes or you can use this proven recipe, which is a two-in-one lotion and sunblock skin product. You can modify the recipe according to your preference, any time.

In this recipe, you would need the following ingredients:

0.5 ounce pure beeswax

4 ounces of grape seed oil

4 ounces of distilled water

10 drops of Rosemary Extract (if not available, Vitamin E T-50 oil can be used) -this is the preservative

15 drops of any essential oil (this is optional)

Non-nano sized zinc oxide powder - the amount will vary according to the SPF that you want. Here is the guide.

Preferred SPF	% of non-nano sized zinc oxide powder
o Low SPF (2-5)	5%
o Moderate SPF (6-11)	10%
o High SPF (12-19)	15%
o Ultra High SPF (more than 20)	20%

* This measurement is based on the overall weight of the lotion. For instance, if your lotion weighs 8 ounces and you want SPF 10, add 0.8 ounces of non-nano sized zinc oxide powder. Observe proper safety measures when handling zinc oxide powder.

Directions:

1. Melt the beeswax with the grape seed oil on a thick-bottomed pot, Pour the melted beeswax into a mason jar that has a wide mouth. Set aside to cool.
2. In another clean container, combine the following ingredients but make sure first that they are not too warm to too cold. They must have the same temperature as the room temperature. These are the rosemary oil, water, (or the Vitamin E T-50) and essential oil. This is the water-rosemary mixture. Set aside.
3. Using a stick blender, pour the water-rosemary mixture slowly into the wax and oil mixture. Blend constantly for 3 to 5 minutes. Make sure that the mixture emulsifies.
4. At this point, observe safety precaution by wearing protective apparel like gloves, facemask and eye goggles. Add zinc oxide powder depending on your desired SPF level and sprinkle into the mix using a fork or a small whisk. Mix well. Small lumps may appear.

Just let it sit for 24 hours and that will cause the zinc oxide to soften. The color should be a slight grey. Then, mix again.

5. Store the finished product in a sealed container. This can last up to 2 months. Placing it in the refrigerator can prolong shelf life.

That's it! You have a lotion that can help keep your skin soft and smooth plus a sunscreen that can protect you from harmful rays and skin cancer. Use this non-greasy lotion every time you will be exposed to the sun, especially any time from 10 am to 3pm. This is not waterproof so if you are going to swim or if you perspire a lot, reapply frequently.

Also, you can help maintain that healthy skin by avoiding the harmful rays of the sun as much as you can. After all, prevention is really better than cure.

Chapter 9: Toxic ingredients That You Should Not Use

There are some ingredients that can help your homemade lotion to emulsify, thicken, last longer, or have that consistent smoothness. However, some of these ingredients have some toxic side effects that can harm your skin. Your homemade lotions would be better off without them.

Here is the list of ingredients to avoid

- Alkyloamides. By themselves, alkyloamides are not toxic. However, when combined with nitrosamines, they turn carcinogenic. Although they are known as thickening agents, emulsifiers and emollients in lotion, try to complete your recipes without them. Examples of alkyloamides are:

- DEA or diethanolamides. They are foaming agents and act as emulsifiers. They are formed from fatty acids and diethanolamine.

- MEA or monoethanolamides. These are organic compound that smell like ammonia. They are also popular as cosmetic and lotion ingredients for their emulsifying action.

- TEA or triethanolamides. These have three alcohol groups, making them a strong base. It could add shelf life to the homemade lotions however adverse reactions were reported.

- MIPA or monoisopropanolamides. These act as softener and emulsifier.

- PEG or ethoxylated alkyloamides. These can help stabilize the lotion plus also they act as emulsifier. Still, they are not to be added to your homemade lotions as they are also considered as irritants to the skin.

- Alcohol. Known for its preservative power, alcohol is widely used in making lotions too. Nevertheless, your lotion is better off without it as it can also damage skin by stripping it of its natural acid mantle. This leaves the skin vulnerable to molds, bacteria, viruses, carcinogens, and other toxins. It also dries skin and causes premature aging of the skin.

- Aminomethyl Propanol. This is used to adjust the pH of the lotion. It has been found to be toxic to some organs, like the kidneys and liver, and can cause disruption in the endocrine and nervous systems.

- Borax. The whitening and preservative properties of borax plus its being organic have made this chemical very popular in the manufacture of cosmetic and skin care products. In addition, it is a good buffer, stabilizing the alkalinity or acidity of a solution. However, various studies have linked borax to medical conditions such as cancer, reproductive difficulties, organ problems, and genetic birth defects. Therefore, as a safety precaution, do not add Borax in your homemade lotion.

- Phthalates. Sometimes known as fragrance, phthalates belong to a family of chemical plasticizers. Not only do they make your products smell good but they can moisturize the skin as well. The down side, however, is that they can cause birth defects, liver damage, and reproductive impairments, as observed during experiments with lab animals. Hence, the possibility of affecting the human the same way cannot be eliminated. In most instances, products with phthalates were reported to cause headaches, nausea, dizziness, and some respiratory problems among the users.

- Glycols. These are actually considered as safe so long as the amount would not exceed 5% of the total amount of the lotion. Excess amounts can lead to birth defects, kidney and liver damages, and contact dermatitis. They are used as humectants in lotions. Never put glycols when you are making your lotion into sunscreen. The glycol family includes the following: propylene glycol, carbitol, glycerin, ethylene glycol, and diethylene glycol.

Your homemade lotion can have the feel, the thickness, the consistency, and the longer shelf life with just the use of all natural and safe ingredients. At the same time, these natural ingredients are environment-friendly. By making your own lotion, you do not only ensure the safety of your own and of other users' skin but have contributed to the safety of the environment as well.

Chapter 10: How To Troubleshoot Problems In Your Homemade Lotion

Many factors affect the outcomes of your lotion. That is why it sometimes takes a lot of experiments before one could perfect a lotion recipe. A single deviation from your recipe could end up into a mess. However, do not be disheartened. A simple tweak could save you from repeating the process and wasting all those ingredients.

Here are the seven common problems being encountered when making your own lotion. Learn how you can troubleshoot these problems easily.

1. The lotion is too thin. When you apply it on your skin, it seems as if you are putting on liquid instead of a lotion. Instead of feeling soft and smooth, your skin feels wet and nothing else. The problem occurs because of excess water. This is easy enough to fix. It simply needs recalculation of the percentages of the ingredients plus a reduction in the amount of water.

2. The lotion is too thick. Have you experienced applying a lotion so thick that it requires a lot of effort and time just to apply it? This is the opposite problem of number one. Hence, the solution is simply doing the reverse of number one. This time, increase the percentage of distilled water and recalculate all the percentages of the rest of the ingredients.

3. The lotion is too greasy. With this problem, you can do several things to remedy it. First, you can add tapioca starch together with the additives at the end of the process. This could be tricky but with some practice,

one can remove the greasiness and have the appropriate feel and smoothness instead.

Another remedy is to change the oil that you are using. You could try the following oils instead: apricot kernel, fractioned coconut oil, sweet almond, jojoba, or macadamia nut. Be careful though that you and the other recipients of the lotions are not allergic to nuts. The last option is to add isopropyl miristate (IPM). Although IPM is not an organic and natural ingredient, it is not sensitizing also. It could make your lotion have a dry, velvety emollient feel to it. Add less than 1% of this ingredient as part of the additives in your recipe.

4. The lotion's color is too greyish or murky. This occurs because of the combination of oils and butters. As a rule, darker ingredients would result to dark colored lotions. Replace some of those dark colored ingredients with light colored ones such as clear jojoba or fractioned coconut oil. Using rosemary extract powder or oil will give you a greenish tint. For most users, this is not an issue as this hue is well accepted. If you think the lotion is perfect except for the color and it doesn't bother you at all, then it's all right to use. However, if you are going to give it as a gift, the recipient might think that it is not fresh or new anymore. You can explain why this is so but it would really be better to just give the lotion with the right color.

5. The texture of the lotion is not smooth. The usual culprit with this problem is the preservative. If the preservative is added with the wrong temperature, the adverse effect is obvious with the texture after the process. There would be this "grainy" rough feel.

The suggestion is to cool down the water to 140 degrees before adding the preservative. Add the oil phase next. Take note that the oil phase should have the same temperature as the water mixture. For some preservatives though, doing this does not solve the problem. It could also be because the mixture was not well mixed or blended. Shea butter is named as the top reason for the rough feel of the lotion due to improper mixing or blending. Use of a gadget to do the mixing or faster mixing of the shea butter sometimes does the trick.

6. The lotion feels too waxy. This happens when ingredients such as stearic acid are added to create a lotion that has more body. In the place of stearic acid, you can use cocoa butter or shea instead. To have a more slippery feel to the skin, you can also add silicone oils to the recipe. These may not be all natural but they can do the trick without the negative effects of skin sensitivity or reactions, as they are not sensitizing. Dimethicone and cyclomethicone can also be added to give that smooth feel. Remember to add the maximum amount of just 1% only. Another solution is to cut back on your emulsifier.

7. The lotion has separated. This means that half part (upper) is watery while the bottom part is thick. The problem might have been the result of adding improper amount of polawax. Read the instruction carefully of how much polawax to add. Another possible reason is temperature problem. Remember that you are supposed to add the oil and water phases when they have the same temperature already. Do not worry. You can still save this lotion.

Just reheat the emulsion gently, preferably in a double broiler. Constantly stir it until it becomes liquid-like again. This time, check the temperature carefully. If the temperature is less than 140 degrees, do not add the preservative yet. Heat it some more. If the temperature is more than 140 degrees, then cool it down first until it reaches the required temperature before you add in the preservatives. Mix well. If you have a high shear mixing device, then this could help you achieve the correct amount of blending. Do this until the emulsion cools and after it stabilizes.

Even if the lotions are not that perfect, you can still use them. Also, make sure that you record everything you do so that you know what works and what do not. Do this until you finally get the correct recipe. Lotion making is fun and easy. However, being patient is a must for simple problems are bound happen.

Chapter 11: DIY Body Lotion Cubes For Kids

Having great skin is not for adults only. Skin care for children is also a must. One is never too young to start caring for the skin and having glowing, youthful, and vibrant skin. However, most parents are hesitant to use commercially prepared baby skin care products. Most of them have experienced their kids having sensitivities or reactions to these products. Why do these things happen?

There are many commercially prepared baby skin care products being sold that actually have ingredients that are too strong for the children's sensitive skin. Instead of making your kids skin healthy, they can even start breakouts and other irritations. The beauty of doing your own body lotion cubes for your kids is that you are very sure of what they are made of. You can have skin products that are free of preservatives and other toxic ingredients.

Another reason children neglect caring for their skin is because they find it boring to apply lotions. That is, unless these lotions are shaped into cubes that look like different animals such as fishes, turtles, birds, lions, to name just a few. Lotions can also take the shape of cars, stars, hearts, letters, flowers, and every shape that you can think of. Plus, they can come in different colors. This is body lotion in cubes. This makes skin care fun for kids.

How can you make body lotion cubes for your kids, for other kids, or for your business?

Involve the children in their skin care. For starters, let the children pick the designs of the molds. This way, they will look forward to using their body lotion cubes. If you do not have molds yet, you can use the regular ice trays. If you are artistic enough, you can cut these cubes into different designs too. Do not use these ice trays for anything else though except for your lotion cubes.

Start with a little amount on your first try. The big kids can do the measurement of the ingredients. Just supervise them so that they will get the perfect amount. However, when it is time to cook the recipe, the adults should do it to avoid accident and burns.

Here is one recipe that even your kids can help you with.

The ingredients are half cup of beeswax, sweet almond oil and shea butter plus 15 drops of any essential oil that you prefer (this is optional). You would need a double broiler (or improvise one) because beeswax is highly flammable and it cannot stand direct heat. To melt the beeswax faster, grate it into smaller pieces.

In a double broiler, heat the water under the broiler until it reaches nearly boiling point temperature. Be careful that you do not get water on your top pot. Doing so could ruin your recipe. When the bottom pot is steaming hot, pour the beeswax on the top pot. Stir until the beeswax starts to melt.

When the beeswax is slightly melted, add the half-cup sweet almond oil. Stir continually until the beeswax is thoroughly melted. This is the time to add in the shea butter. This is the tricky part as shea butter is a little bit "finicky". It has the tendency to turn grainy when the temperature is too high or if it is too long. You have to wait until the end before you heat it up and take note that it melts really fast, so you also have to be fast. Stir thoroughly.

When the shea butter is completely melted, remove the pot from heat. Pour into the molds before the mixture starts to cool and sets in. Here is another tricky part. During the cooling time but before the mixture sets in, drop the essential oil and stir with a toothpick. Do not wait too long or else, it would be too late. You can leave the molds on the table for fifteen minutes or if your kids cannot wait longer, place them on the freezer and in no time at all, the body lotion cubes would be ready. Just pop out the cubes like you would do with regular ice. If you try to bring them out using a knife, the design might be chipped.

The kids would be excited to see the colorful and beautiful designs. For them, it is equivalent to another toy. Instruct them to rub these lotion cubes on their skin, especially on the thick-skinned parts, such as elbows, knees, ankles, and hands. As it touches the skin, it will start to melt a little. This is surely one way of having fun while having glowing and healthy skin among children.

Store the remaining body lotion cubes in an airtight container. Place them in a cool dry place or inside the refrigerator. The kids could get one cube once or twice a day. If you also plan to give them away as gifts, place them in mini jars. Decorate the jar, put a card and that's it. You have a cute, skin care product as a gift that any kid would love to receive.

Making body lotion cubes is fun and easy. Take note however that this is not for kids only. Young and old alike would also enjoy receiving cute body lotion cubes as gifts. You could personalize the gifts by giving them lotion cubes with their name's initials. It is also a great souvenir item to be given during parties, reunions or family gatherings. Plus, they make good promotional items to advertise your store, other business or company.

Lotion cubes are also convenient to bring. Just place them in airtight plastic during travels when liquids are not allowed plus they are less messy. You can take one every time you feel the need to moisture your skin. That is not all. Body lotion cubes or even plain lotions could lead to great profits, too. Find out in the next chapter.

Chapter 12 Homemade Lotion: An Income Generating Hobby

Creating and using your own homemade lotion is not only good for your skin. It is also good for your pockets. Yes, there is a profit to be gained when you turn this hobby into business. Do you know that in 2011, natural and organic beauty products, lotions included, earned a total of $9 billion? The predicted sale for 2015 is at $14 billion. Why is this happening even when the economy is down? This is because more and more people are concern with how they look and how healthy their skin is. They are willing to spend and invest in skin products just to have that glowing and vibrant skin.

If you want to venture into this business but you are having doubts, cheer up. This business has a great potential in bringing you financial gains. Your market is very wide. It includes basically everybody. The young and the old, male or female, rich or poor people – everybody needs and wants good skin.

Plus, this business is easy to do and very safe too. Anybody can do it, whether one is educated or not. Another good thing about this business is it only requires minimal capital to start. There is no need to buy expensive equipment, and the ingredients are cheap. You would not need to rent a space to make and pack those lotions, too. You can do it in the comfort of your kitchen. You do not need to have a store and salespeople to sell them. You can start with just you as both the employer and the employee.

You can do the business without the high cost of advertisement. You can do it online or through word of mouth. When people know that your products are all natural, cheaper and better than the commercially prepared lotions, it would not be long before they share this news to their relative and other friends. You can expect those orders to come in especially during Christmas or Thanksgiving.

Even if the worst scenario comes, which is having poor or little sale of lotions, you have still not lost. You can use them personally. You can give away these lotions to your friends and family members as gifts. You would never run out of ideas where to use these lotions.

How to start a lotion making business

Here are some things you need to do before you start that lotion business.

1. First, get legal.

There are different business plan licensing requirements for each city, estate or country. Become familiar with them and comply with all the requirements. Take note that lotions fall under the Federal Food, Drug and Cosmetic Act. Your lotions do not need to undergo lab tests in order for them to be approved. The only time that you would need to present lab results is when you claim something about your lotions. For instance, saying that it can heal or prevent a specific skin disease, is not allowed without valid proofs. Also, make sure that the additives that you put into your lotions are FDA approved. Part of being legal is obtaining liability insurance as a form of protection for yourself and your business in case an untoward incident arises with regard to your homemade lotion.

2. Prepare your supplies and space.

If you are single, living alone, and have limited space, then your kitchen can be your makeshift office, factory, shop, and storage area, all in one. However, if you have pets or little children, find a different spot in your home where you can keep your supplies and ingredients safely. There should be shelves with locks for the supplies to be stored in just to have added safety in case pets or children happen to go into that spot.

You would need mixing containers and tools to measure the ingredients. For your basic ingredients, you would save a lot of money when you buy in bulk. The same thing applies when you buy special ingredients such as herbs, scents and dried flowers. Bottles, jars or other containers are also being sold by bulk. Among all the ingredients, do not scrimp on lotion base. You would need a stabilized lotion base. This would keep your lotion's shelf life longer. In case you decide to make your own lotion base, put it in the refrigerator to keep it fresh for several months.

3. Create labels.

In creating labels, there are also FDA requirements that you need to know and comply with. Make sure that you have that covered. For instance, it is a must that all ingredients that you used in your lotion are listed in the label. Also, instructions on how to use the lotion should be included.

Another FDA requirement is that your company's name, address and contact numbers should also be a part of the label. Do not claim anything about your lotion or put false statements about your products as this can backfire against you. This is a form of false advertising. Unsubstantiated claims are prohibited. Check if there are other FDA requirements as they differ from each city, estate and country. After complying with all the FDA regulations, then you can design your label the way you want it to. This is important as most people make the label as the deciding factor before buying a product, especially if it is their first time to buy that product. Afterwards, they buy again or reorder because of the quality of the product. Make the label attractive and catchy.

4. Determine the price of the lotion.

This is also an important factor to consider so that potential buyers would support your products than their previous products. If you can offer lower or the same price as their usual products, then the chance of them buying your products is higher. Compute the basic expenses like the cost of ingredients, electricity or gas, supplies, labels and packaging expenses, taxes, and even your time in making the lotion. Add the profit margin, again taking heed of the prices of other similar and more popular products.

5. Start marketing and selling.

You can do this in several ways to ensure higher financial gains. Aside from giving away small samples to your friends, neighbors, coworkers, and anybody you know and even to strangers, you can also start advertising in all your social media accounts. Use your account in Twitter, Facebook, Instagram, and Tumbler, among others to advertise your products. These are free and very effective means of reaching potential clients.

You can also set up an ecommerce website so that you would be able to reach more people. In addition, you can look for shops, boutiques or even your local grocery stores that would be willing to carry your products in exchange for some percentage with the sales or as whatever you agreed upon.

You can also offer discounts and other promos when clients buy or order in bulk. Or have a loyalty card that would earn points or small items every time the client buys from you. Later on, they can use those points when they buy products from you again. Consider expanding your business by renting a space and selling from there. Though print ads are expensive, they can be effective too. You may want to consider that strategy in the future.

Lastly, there may be other interested businessmen who would like to franchise your store or products. In this way, you do not only earn from the franchise but your products or stores get to be set up in different parts of the country or even the world.

6. Be adventurous.

Create different types of lotions. Clients are always on the look out for something new and different. If you are hesitant, try to make small samples first so as to test the waters. If the new products become a hit, then that is the time that you can make them in bigger bottles. Do your assignment and research the latest fad in lotions all over the world. Find out what people are buying. Cater to the needs of the children by coming up with new and exciting designs of lotion cubes. Continue to look for updates and watch out for new trends and products from your competitions.

7. Ask for feedback.

Be open for both positive and negative feedbacks to improve your business. Be the main critique of your own product. Try all your products so that you have first-hand assessment of how good or bad your products are.

Lotions are very helpful in making your skin healthy, soft, and vibrant. Today, start your journey to a healthy skin through using homemade lotions. They are not only safer and economical but they can even be the start of something profitable for you.

Conclusion

Thank you again for purchasing this book!

I hope this book was able to help you learn the things you need to know in making natural homemade lotion.

The next step is to apply what you have learned and create your own lotion.

Finally, if you enjoyed this book, please take the time to share your thoughts and post a review on Amazon. We do our best to reach out to readers and provide the best value we can. Your positive review will help us achieve that. It'd be greatly appreciated!

Thank you and good luck!

Check Out My Other Books

Below you'll find some of my other popular books that are popular on Amazon and Kindle as well. Simply click on the links below to check them out. Alternatively, you can visit my author page on Amazon to see other work done by me.

Coconut Oil for Skin Care & Hair Loss

http://amzn.to/1p0GwGC

Coconut Oil & Weight Loss for Beginners

http://amzn.to/1jqdy3R

Walk Your Way To Weight Loss

http://amzn.to/1jOHpgy

Quick Easy Healthy Snack Ideas for Kids

http://amzn.to/1grvURn

Oil Pulling for Beginners

http://amzn.to/SBDoXb

Healing Babies & Children With Aromatherapy For Beginners

http://amzn.to/TOHJHs

Carb Cycling for Fast Easy Weight Loss

http://amzn.to/THn8Vl

Beauty Products for Beginners

http://amzn.to/1nVvwNw

Body Lotions for Beginners

http://amzn.to/S3XlWh

Container Gardening for Beginners

http://amzn.to/1oLb2p0

Vegetable Gardening for beginners

http://amzn.to/1lqCCIK

Raised Bed Gardening for beginners

http://amzn.to/1nHY0ry

Greenhouse Gardening for beginners

http://amzn.to/UEmOr2

Companion Gardening for beginners

http://amzn.to/1hYzeEl

Essential Oils Box Set #1 Healing Babies and Children With Aromatherapy for Beginners & Oil Pulling for Beginners

http://amzn.to/1yZoH0Q

Essential Oils Box Set #2 Carb Cycling For Fast Easy Weight Loss + Walk Your Way to Weight Loss

http://amzn.to/Tu5xiL

Essential Oils Box Set #3 Beauty Products For Beginners + Body Lotions For Beginners

http://amzn.to/1qnVLNQ

Essential Oils Box Set #4 Coconut Oil & Weigh Loss for Beginners & Coconut Oil for Skin Care & Hair Loss

http://amzn.to/1iQQUlN

Essential Oils Box Set #5 Coconut Oil Skin Care & Hair Loss + Healing Babies & Children & Aromatherapy for Beginners + Beauty Products for Beginners +Body Lotions For Beginners +Oil Pulling for Beginners

http://amzn.to/1qGPc6D

Essential Oils Box Set #6Carb Cycling for Fast Easy Weight Loss + Oil Pulling Therapy For Beginners + Walk Your Way to Weight Loss + Coconut Oil & Weight for Beginners + Coconut Oil for Skin Care & Hair Loss

http://amzn.to/UXAAoz

Essential Oils Box Set #7 Coconut Oil for Skin Care & Hair Loss + Oil Pulling Therapy For Beginners + Healing Babies and Children with Aromatherapy for Beginners

http://amzn.to/1nUdbg5

Gardening Box Set #1 Raised Bed Gardening For Beginners + Vegetable Gardening For Beginners + Companion Gardening For Beginners + Greenhouse Gardening for Beginners +Container Gardening for Beginners

http://amzn.to/1lZOsse

Gardening Box Set #2 Container Gardening For Beginners + Ultimate Guide to Companion Gardening for Beginners

http://amzn.to/1q4wma5

If the links do not work, for whatever reason, you can simply search for these titles on the Amazon website to find them.

www.ingramcontent.com/pod-product-compliance
Lightning Source LLC
Chambersburg PA
CBHW070622290526
45790CB00002B/951